HOW TO GIVE UP SEX

On your first day giving up sex you are probably feeling a little excited and also a little apprehensive. Can you do it? What if you fail? Will you feel demoralised if you find yourself unable to resist temptation and fall back into your old sexual ways? You feel the odds are all against being successful. After all, there are so many things working against you – you're attractive, interesting and have often been given reason to believe you are a great lover.

Don't worry. It's not as difficult as it seems. In the first place, you are probably not as attractive as you think – or as interesting. And as for being a great lover, this is almost certainly imagined. A partner may have whispered this to you once or twice, but what about all the times when they didn't? *Why* didn't they? Perhaps you were painfully bad, even useless? There is certainly room for optimism.

The good news about celibacy is that you have probably been practising it for years without even knowing. Every time you said you had a headache, were too tired or couldn't get it together you were in fact being celibate. Or you may have thought you were having sex but your partner thought you were being celibate. One way or the other, you are likely to have spent more of your life celibate than not – this is something to build on.

About the Authors

Apart from a few minor slip-ups Roger Planer and Richard McBrien have been celibate for well over a week. Over this period they have established a reputation as two of the most innovative celibates of their generation, between them amassing a vast amount of experience which is mounting all the time.

Both authors have been celibate with most of the major figures of their time and their names continue to be linked with many more. Their only regret is that so many slipped through the net in the early days.

Other books by the same authors include 'Behind Open Doors – Who's been celibate with Who in Hollywood' and 'Celibacy and Semiotics, a Deconstructionist Approach'.

Between writing and lecture commitments the authors now spend most of their time being celibate with a growing band of admirers. Neither are happily married or live in Surrey.

How To Give Up Sex

Roger Planer
and
Richard McBrien

with illustrations by Jon Riley

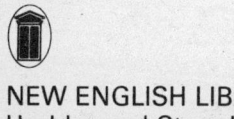

NEW ENGLISH LIBRARY
Hodder and Stoughton

Copyright © 1989 by
Roger Planer & Richard McBrien

Illustration copyright © 1989 by
Jon Riley

First published in Great Britain in
1989 by New English Library
Paperbacks

A New English Library
paperback original

*The characters and situations in this
book are entirely imaginary and
bear no relation to any real person
or actual happenings.*

This book is sold subject to the
condition that it shall not, by way
of trade or otherwise, be lent,
re-sold, hired out or otherwise
circulated without the publishers
prior consent in any form of
binding or cover other than that in
which it is published and without
a similar condition including this
condition being imposed on the
subsequent purchaser.

No part of this publication may
be reproduced or transmitted in
any form or by any means,
electronically or mechanically,
including photocopying, recording
or any information storage or
retrieval system, without either
the prior permission in writing
from the publisher or a licence,
permitting restricted copying. In the
United Kingdom such licences are
issued by the Copyright Licensing
Agency, 33–34 Alfred Place,
London WC1E 7DP.

British Library C.I.P.

Planer, Roger
 How to give up sex.
 1. Celibacy
 I. Title II. McBrien, Richard
 306.7'32

 ISBN 0-450-49473-X

Printed and bound in Great Britain
for Hodder and Stoughton
Paperbacks, a division of Hodder
and Stoughton Limited, Mill Road,
Dunton Green, Sevenoaks, Kent
TN13 2YA. (Editorial Office:
47 Bedford Square, London
WC1B 3DP) by Richard Clay Limited,
Bungay, Suffolk. Photoset
by Rowland Phototypesetting
Limited, Bury St Edmunds, Suffolk.

FOREWORD

The History of Celibacy

There was very little to do in the Garden of Eden. Had God provided a few more diversions, some decent restaurants, an amusement arcade, the whole question of sex might never have arisen. As it was, Adam and Eve had nothing better to do than listen to a talking snake and willingly go along with whatever crazy idea came into its head. Had there been a decent continental holiday on offer things might have worked out differently. But once the idea of sex had been introduced successive generations went on doing it simply out of ignorance and boredom.

Despite rigorous attempts to repress the efforts and achievements of celibates, it is possible to trace a resistance to the overwhelming sexual trend. The innate tendency of

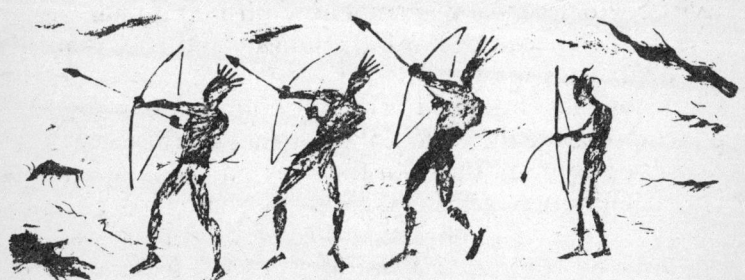

'Homo Non-Erectus' or 'Celibate Pit Man' discovered in the cave drawings of Northern France

celibate communities to peter out after one generation has made it difficult to chart their progress accurately, but recent archaelogical evidence points to the emergence of Homo Non-Erectus as long ago as 5000 years before Christ.

In the seventeenth century, the first stirrings of celibate literature were vigorously suppressed by Royal Decree. A Kama Sutra for Celibates, compiled *'for thofe reluctant to fornicate'* and listing over a hundred now lost positions for celibates, was burned in the streets, condemned by the Church for *'not being in the leaft bit bawdy or ribald'*. Gangs of vigilantes were often seen rounding up celibate suspects and many widows and single folk, unjustly accused of not having sex, were killed or imprisoned in mixed cells.

Reasons for the brutal suppression and ridicule of celibates remained obscure until the early twentieth century when the advent of psychoanalysis for the first time revealed a deep-rooted desire in us all not to have sex. It is the repression of this latent yearning for celibacy which causes most neuroses.

According to theory, the baby starts life as a celibate being and longs to get back to this original state. At around three years it experiences a strong desire to talk to its father and not have sex with its mother – this is the start of a healthy celibate life.

During childhood an experience such as stumbling across one's parents not having sex can have a deep and traumatic effect. In later life this may result in intense feelings of guilt every time one is celibate, leading to the conviction that celibacy is somehow dirty and shameful. These memories can be hard to eradicate and may require years of analysis to overcome.

Only now, late into the twentieth century, are we beginning to appreciate the effects of these theoretical advances. The old 'uptight' attitudes of the previous generation are finally beginning to relax and a new permissiveness about celibacy is entering public consciousness. Ordinary people who don't want to have sex or are 'just not feeling like it at the moment' are speaking up for themselves, unafraid of being labelled 'abnormal' by the rest of society. At last it is possible to foresee a time when celibacy will be universally enjoyed without guilt or secrecy and sex will finally be put back in the closet where it belongs.

It would take too long to list all the people who have helped with this book by not having sex with the authors. But we would like to take this opportunity to thank them all for their invaluable support. Without their tireless and insistent rebuttals this book would not have been possible.

CONTENTS

Introduction	xiii
GIVING UP SEX	1
Early Days	3
Bad Sex for Beginners	5
Foreplay	9
Getting Down to It	15
Orgasms	21
Towards Celibacy	23
THE JOY OF CELIBACY	25
The Joy of Celibacy	26
Preparation	27
Being Celibate for the First Time	31
Celibacy and the Single Person	41
The Facts About Celibacy	47
Adjusting to Celibate Life	51
Spicing Up Your Celibate Life	55
The Future	63

INTRODUCTION

The Art of Not Having Sex

Like driving a car or making a fire, being celibate is something everyone thinks they can do naturally. Even practised celibates sometimes react fiercely to the suggestion that there is anything they don't already know about the subject.

The fact is there is a great deal more to celibacy than just 'not having sex'. More and more people are discovering they have an almost limitless capacity for celibate experience. Indeed, it is our ability to enjoy the rich variety of celibate life that distinguishes us from the animals.

It is not the intention of this book to provide a set of 'rules' for celibates, to dictate how and when, or indeed with whom, you should be celibate. Rather we hope that by discussing the pleasures and pitfalls of celibacy frankly and without shame we can open your eyes and enable you to lead a rewarding, guilt-free celibate life.

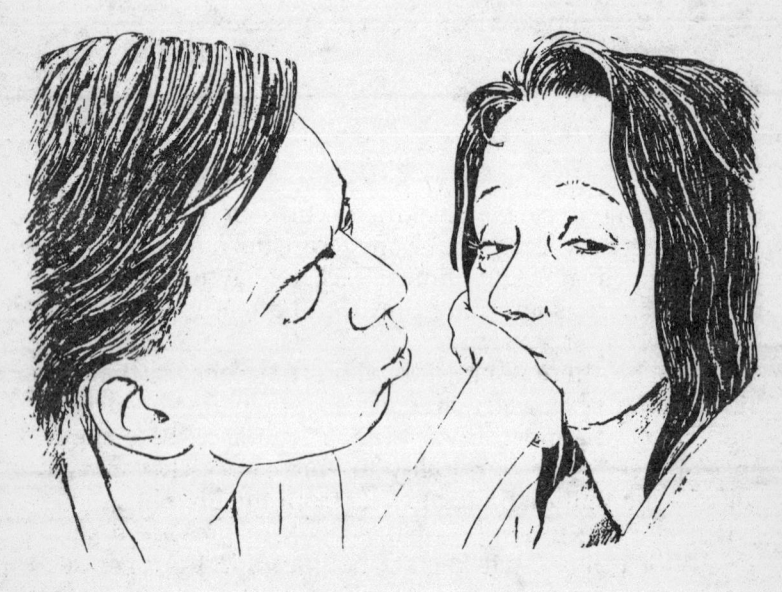

Giving Up Sex

EARLY DAYS

On your first day giving up sex you are probably feeling a little excited and also a little apprehensive. Can you do it? What if you fail? Will you feel demoralised if you find yourself unable to resist temptation and fall back into your old sexual ways? You feel the odds are all against being successful. After all, there are so many things working against you – you're attractive, interesting and have often been given reason to believe you are a great lover.

Don't worry. It's not as difficult as it seems. In the first place, you are probably not as attractive as you think – or as interesting. And as for being a great lover, this is almost certainly imagined. A partner may have whispered this to you once or twice, but what about all the times when they didn't? *Why* didn't they? Perhaps you were painfully bad, even useless? There is certainly room for optimism.

The good news about celibacy is that you have probably been practising it for years without even knowing. Every time you said you had a headache, were too tired or couldn't get it together you were in fact being celibate. Or you may have thought you were having sex but your partner thought you were being celibate. One way or the other, you are likely to have spent more of your life celibate than not – this is something to build on.

Telling your partner

Although you can't wait to start being celibate, you may be reluctant to break the news to your partner; will they share your enthusiasm? Sooner or later you will have to tell them, so it's much better to come straight out with it than let them discover it for themselves. After all, it's difficult to be celibate with a partner who's still having sex with you.

Naturally a number of questions will arise, so it is as well to be prepared with some convincing answers.

Some typical questions your partner will ask:

If we stop having sex together can I have sex with someone else?
   No. Explain that not only are you not going to have sex together but neither of you is going to have sex with anyone else.

Does being celibate mean not being in love?
   It is quite possible to be in love and still be celibate, though obviously some of the most successful celibate relationships have been between people who dislike each other.

Are you being celibate with me so you can save your sexual energies for casual friends and acquaintances?
   It's vital that you establish an atmosphere of mutual trust at this point if you're going to explore your celibate potential together. Remember, you are not so much giving up sex as taking up celibacy.

Can we just be celibate when we're not having sex?
   Yes, at first. Most successful celibates start on this part-time basis and gradually extend the periods between sex until they enjoy continual abstinence.

BAD SEX FOR BEGINNERS

How often should I be celibate?

Do not get carried away by your enthusiasm and try to cut out all sex immediately. If you do, you will simply smoulder for a week and then go at it so hard for a month you won't be able to walk. First you must concentrate on making sex a lot more disappointing. Without a poor and unsatisfactory sex life to look back on you are unlikely ever to be a fulfilled celibate. It may take several months of concentrated effort, but once you have built a firm base of poor sex you will both be itching to get home to not have sex together.

How difficult will it be?

Easier for some than for others, this depends largely on the quality of your current sex life. Some couples have to work at 'bad sex' for months and only succeed in making it fairly average. Others may be delighted to discover they have a natural aptitude for it and have been practising it for most of their lives.

First Principles

Take a long hard look at your sex life. Are you attracted to each other? Were you ever attracted to each other? Are you having sex now just to be polite? With a little encouragement could you find each other really quite unattractive?

You may not be able to answer these questions with absolute certainty, years of routine sex having clouded your vision. It's therefore necessary to get back to basics.

The Human Body

Apart from a few doubts you had during adolescence you are probably convinced that the human body is, at least in principle, beautiful. This view has been perpetuated over the years by the tireless insistence of sex educationalists and artists. You may even feel your own body conforms to this ideal – this is an illusion you must overcome.

Exploring your Body

Make sure the room is warm and well-lit, preferably with a fluorescent tube. Pour yourself a couple of stiff drinks to relax and then stand with your partner in front of a mirror. Slowly examine each other's bodies, paying particular attention to blemishes, irregularities and pockmarks. Draw attention to anything you feel is not perfect, from small spots to large areas of flab. The effect on your partner will be considerably enhanced if the expression on your face is critical.

This exercise is amazingly effective at eroding confidence in your appearance. Soon, in your imagination, 'problem areas' will far outweigh good points. You will also find that your tolerance of your partner's appearance was only dependent on their tolerance of yours. Once you have been made aware of your ugly stretch marks you will be less inclined to overlook a hairy paunch.

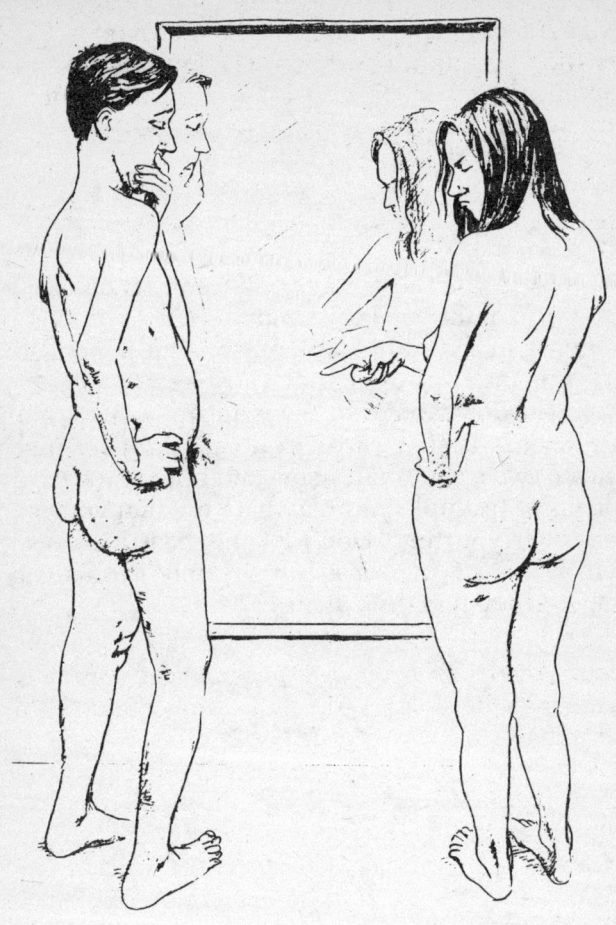

Everybody is NOT beautiful. Beauty is NOT in the eye of the beholder

Talking it Over

During the day try to encourage an atmosphere of free and open exchange in which you can honestly tell each other how you feel. Remember, it is the little things you say to your partner that will keep the relationship on ice. Comments such as 'You look your age today' or 'That's a nasty spot on your nose' will help you both to remain distant. You might also like to coin pet-names for each other which highlight shortcomings and failures, such as 'Mr-Two-Seconds' or 'Bum Flab'. These can be their most effective when used in public.

Hangups

Use the past to your advantage. Concentrate on old sexual hangups and failures. For example, try to remember a time when you did not reach orgasm simultaneously and develop this into a neurosis.

When you do manage to have an uneventful night be sure to discuss it afterwards in detail. Go over just why you found each other unarousing and note down particular turn-offs. For example you may hate it when your partner slobbers over your ear. Don't let this pass but speak up, let them know it's bad or it hurts – only in this way can you ensure they will do it again.

FOREPLAY

Foreplay is one of the secrets of successful sex – it stimulates, excites and prepares you for the full pleasures of love-making. If you feel confident enough by this stage, try doing without it altogether. However, there is an art to making foreplay as unexciting as possible which you might like to try.

Undressing

Experienced celibates know there is a right way to undress to completely sabotage any interest their partners might have in making love.

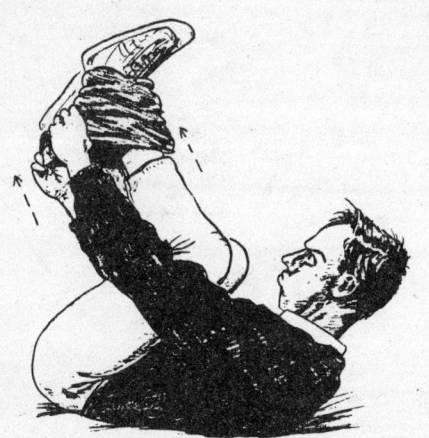

Trousers first – remember to leave socks and shoes on

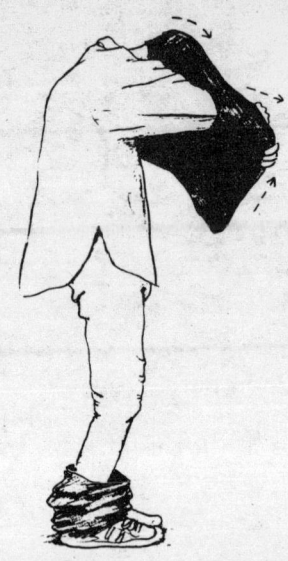

A nice tight neckline can hold things up for hours

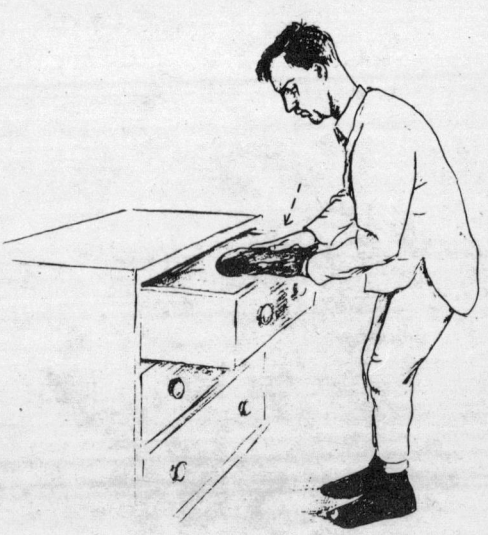

Neatness is often overlooked as an effective turn-off

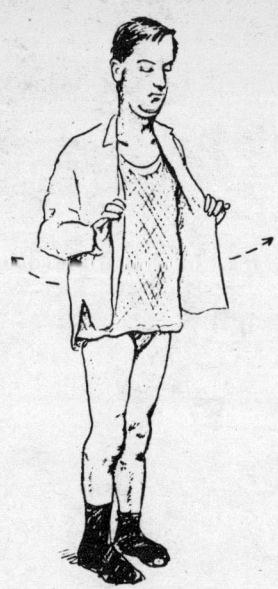

Do not underestimate the unerotic power of the string vest

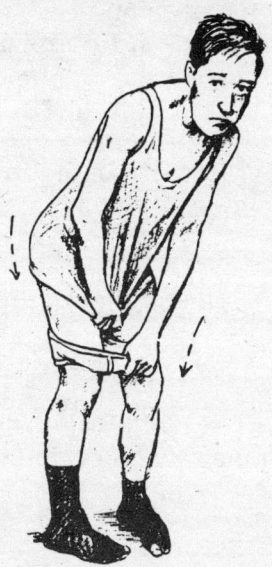

Almost ready for celibacy

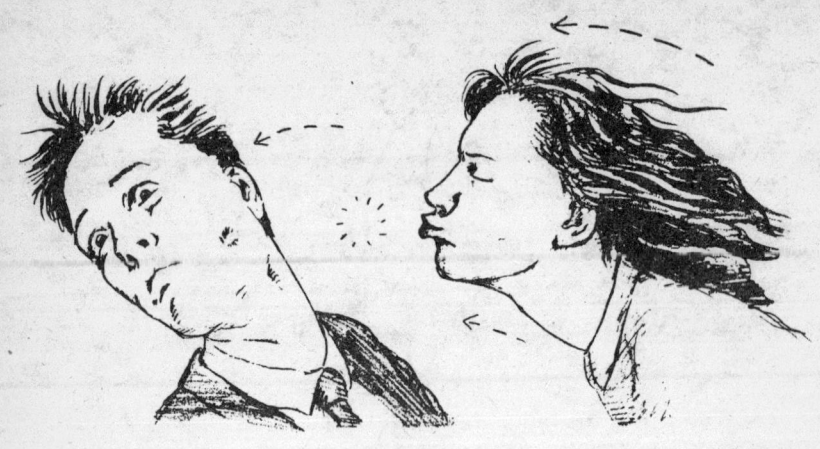

The aggressive kiss-butt can deter the most amorous suitor

Kissing

The universal sign of affection, the lovers' basic tool, the kiss symbolises the care and desire many people feel for each other. For the celibate it offers almost unlimited scope for mishandling. Here are some basic tips:

> Imagine you are entering into combat with an opponent.
> Always keep your lips dry and chapped.
> If possible miss the intended target – this can confuse your partner.
> Be sloppy – open your mouth like a fish, bringing plenty of saliva towards the front with your tongue, then approach the kissee as if you were trying to wet a very large stamp.

Shy and inexperienced bad kissers who fear their efforts may be erotic, can practise on everyday objects about the house, such as a wall, damp sponge or firm omelette.

Specials

You will need to be sensitive to your partner's needs if you are going to know how to ignore them. Discover that special thing your partner finds erotic – then cut it out. Breaking the habit of oral sex is best done by trying to do it only to yourself.

Laughter

Laughter is one of the great joys of celibacy, marking us out from other animals who are just not having sex. It can instantly transform a sexual advance into a celibate one. Perhaps start with a smile when your partner suggests sex, develop this into a snigger as they undress and finally roll around on the floor in hysterics, pointing at them incredulously, saying, 'What, with you?!'

Caressing

Stroking can be lethal to the novice celibate, instilling a warm feeling of well-being and eroticism. If you cannot omit it altogether at least make sure it is as uncomfortable as possible.

Substituting a wire brush for finger-tips dipped in baby-oil can produce extremely unerotic skin sensations. In the absence of a wire-brush grade three sandpaper can be used.

Warning!

Such practices may turn out to be one of your partner's secret fantasies, resulting in an embarrassing bout of sexual fulfilment. It is therefore advisable to introduce them slowly, checking for any adverse reaction – if your partner

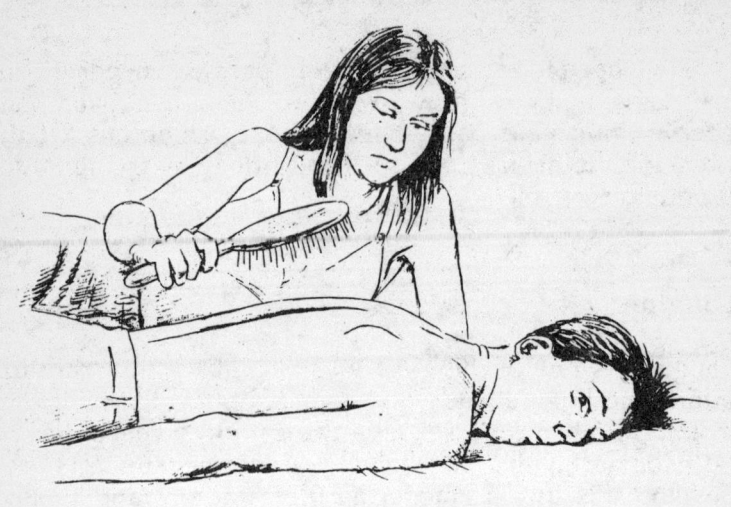

The Wire Brush Off

starts to breathe heavily or sweat profusely stop immediately and take a cold shower together.

Going Off Your Partner

By now you should be experiencing strangely ambivalent feelings towards your partner. When they enter the room you do not feel any different, when they fail to ring up for several days you do not notice. These are all good signs. What you are experiencing is what 'straight sexual' couples call 'going off your partner'. What they fail to appreciate is that this is not the end of a passionate affair but the beginning of something much more significant. It is a tragic fact that thousands of couples have split up just as they were about to discover the delights of celibacy.

GETTING DOWN TO IT

Despite these general feelings of queasiness, you may find your libido is still in control, driving you on in the pursuit of sexual gratification. Once you have confounded these expectations a couple of times the whole thing will become much easier.

Where and When

Confining sexual activities to the bedroom will add a helpful air of monotonous familiarity to your love-making. Double beds should be replaced by bunk beds or a hammock, sheets be made of hessian and duvets exchanged for heavy, military-style blankets.

You might try scheduling sex to rid it of any unwanted element of surprise, comparing diaries several weeks in advance. Alternatively, you can retain spontaneity by choosing a moment when you know your partner will least want to have sex, for example the morning after a late party when you have stale breath and, with luck, little bits of white scum on your mouth. Remember to leave the curtains open so bright sunlight floods in highlighting skin imperfections and wrinkles.

Embarrassment can also be useful. Bad sex is considerably enhanced by a constant fear of being overlooked or overheard. Encourage friends to drop round unexpectedly and always leave doors and windows open so you can be surprised easily.

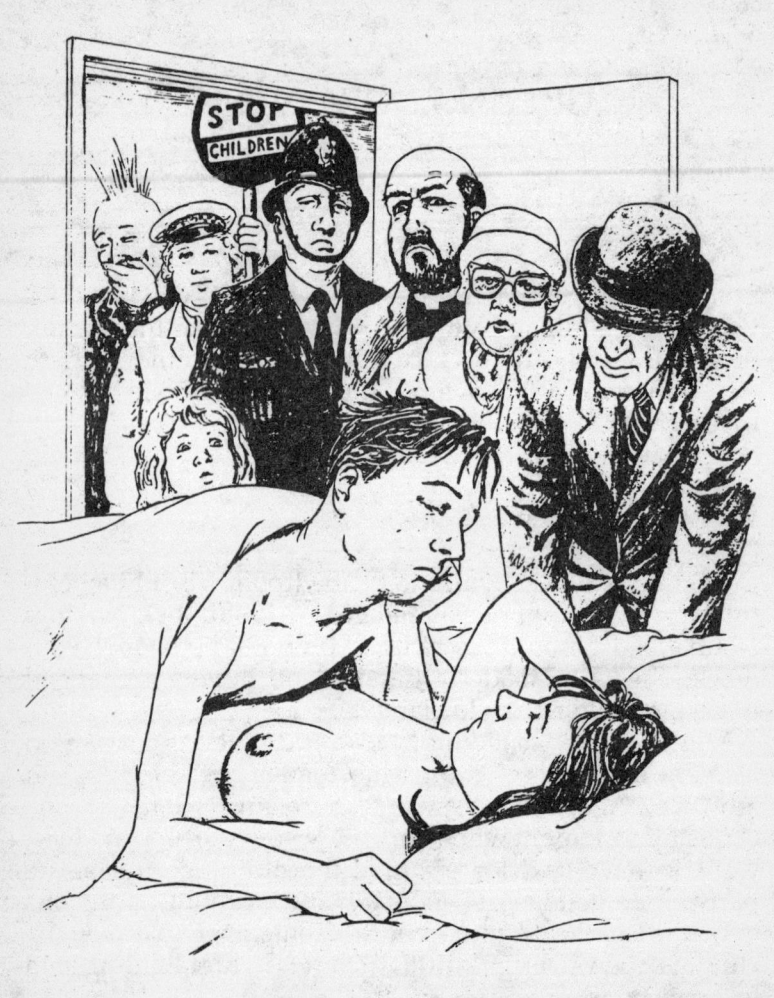

Some couples find an audience a real passion-killer

Positions

For centuries people have been identifying and classifying new positions for making love. As a sexually active person you will naturally have tried many of them with varying degrees of success. Now you can capitalise on all your experience by repeating the most awkward and unsatisfying of them. Once you have found your least favourite position, stick to it. Meanwhile, there are one or two things you can do to make the whole experience more tedious.

Introduce other activities into the sex act. Cleaning the flat while your partner is attempting to arouse you can be a turn-off and also save time with household chores.

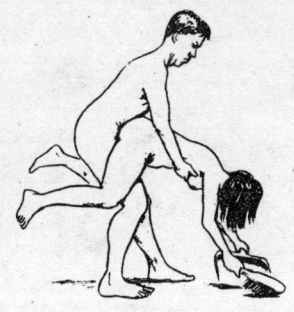

The Wheelbarrow

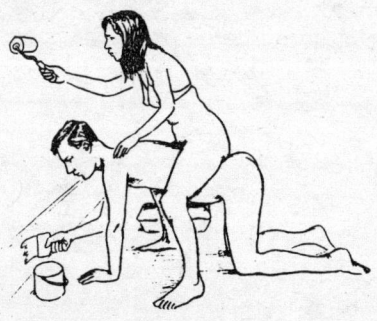

Cowboy Decorating

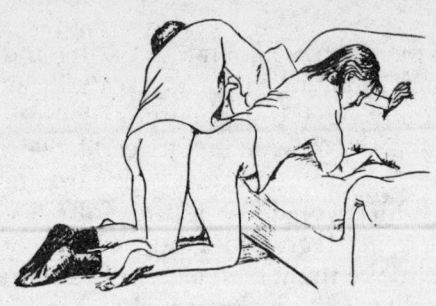

Looking for change down the back of the sofa

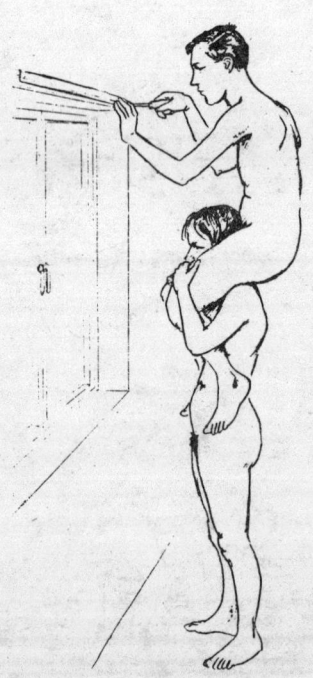

Fitting the Curtain Rail

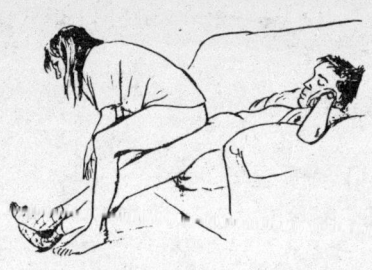
Watching TV

Coitus Interruptus

The emphasis here should be on the interruptus rather than the coitus. The more complicated the position you choose, the less actual sex you will have. If you are precariously balanced on the edge of a shelf and make a mistake, it could be a good few hours before you are at it again – that is a good few hours of 'not having sex'.

Timing

You'll enhance the anti-climactic effect if you try to bring sex to a short and unsatisfactory conclusion. Keep a record of how long you take to make love and try to improve it each time. With practice you may even to shave a few seconds off the all-time record of two-and-a-half seconds.

Talking Clean

What you say to your partner in bed can make all the difference. In moments of extremity some people like to 'talk clean' by shouting out clean words, such as 'Shiny!'

or 'Sparkling!' Others prefer to whisper sweet nothings, like 'What time is it?' or 'I ate a bagel today.'

Marital Aids

Some couples like to use external devices to help their celibacy – the greatest of these being marriage itself. It has a proven track record as a sexual antidote, with over half of all married couples achieving almost total celibacy within the first three years.

Contraception can also help in dampening sexual ardour. Not only does it involve a lot of fumbling in the dark trying to find the right pack, pill or lotion, but the very sight of some prophylactics can be off-putting. These are best arranged in an attractive array by the bedside and produced at the appropriate moment.

Accompany this by a discussion of the side-effects of each method, for example you might like to point out that the pill has a fifteen per cent chance of causing cancer while the IUD can make women sterile.

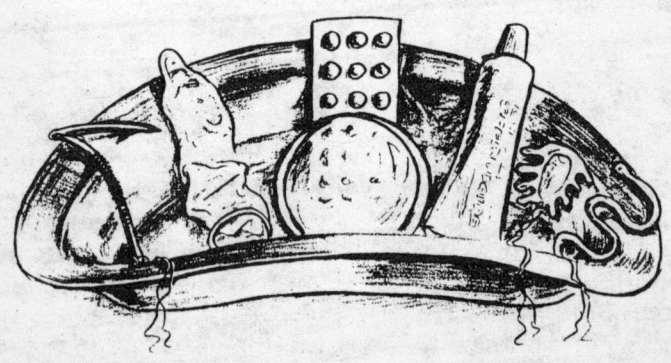

ORGASMS

One of the main worries novice celibates face is when sex drags on for well over a minute giving enormous pleasure to both parties. In 'bad sex' you are at a great advantage if you can make the sacrifice of having a quick orgasm in order to ensure that your partner doesn't have one at all.

Simultaneous Orgasms

After years of practice and perseverance you will be accustomed to experiencing simultaneous orgasms and may find it hard to break the habit. One way to overcome this difficulty is to make your orgasm simultaneous with something other than your partner – for example the State Opening of Parliament or 'Gardeners' Question Time'.

Premature Ejaculation

There is great pressure on the male celibate to experience premature ejaculation as soon as possible – preferably some hours or even weeks before any sexual contact. If this is not achieved there is the danger of bringing the woman to the point of orgasm herself – something she will almost definitely resent however polite she may be at the time.

Premature ejaculation is therefore a major cause of anxiety for those men who can't achieve it. During the sex act, if the man feels he is about to last several hours, fulfilling his partner totally, he should start to think entirely of himself and how nice it would be to get the whole thing over as soon as possible. He should fill his mind with highly stimulating images and concentrate hard on the matter in hand.

Faking It

From time to time most women trying to give up sex suffer the unexpected orgasm. If you are on your own this need be nothing to be ashamed of. If you are with someone else it may be helpful for your partner's sake to fake it and pretend nothing happened as it can be very dispiriting for him to know he's brought you to this point.

TOWARDS CELIBACY

Your dreams will be a good indication of how your subconscious is dealing with the idea of celibacy. You may find, for instance, that you are still dreaming of tunnels but are building rather than going through them. If you do find yourself in a train hurtling towards a tidal wave, concentrate on the celibate aspects of your situation. Complain to the guard about the curtain material used or ask when the buffet car opens.

With experience the imagery may become more explicit. You will start to dream of man-eating vulvas, of giant penises chasing you down the High Street. Uptight sexual activists call these taboos, even neurotic obsessions, but in fact they are signs of a healthy celibate libido expressing itself in your subconscious.

Celibate Drives

As your sex life deteriorates you will become increasingly aware of a burning desire not to have sex. You may have felt this sensation before but never so strongly. Don't worry, it's simply that your celibate drive has been aroused.

Everyone has a different celibate drive – while some just can't get enough and would like to be celibate twenty-four hours a day, others are less demanding and find that the occasional bout of celibacy will satisfy them for some time.

Different celibate drives are upsetting when you are both

trying to give up sex. Some people find they continue to suffer from multiple orgasms while their partners are already achieving a state of complete indifference.

Ideally you should create a situation where sex is equally unsatisfactory for you both, when you can honestly say 'It was terrible for me, too.' Then and only then will you be ready to progress to the joys of celibacy.

The Joy of Celibacy

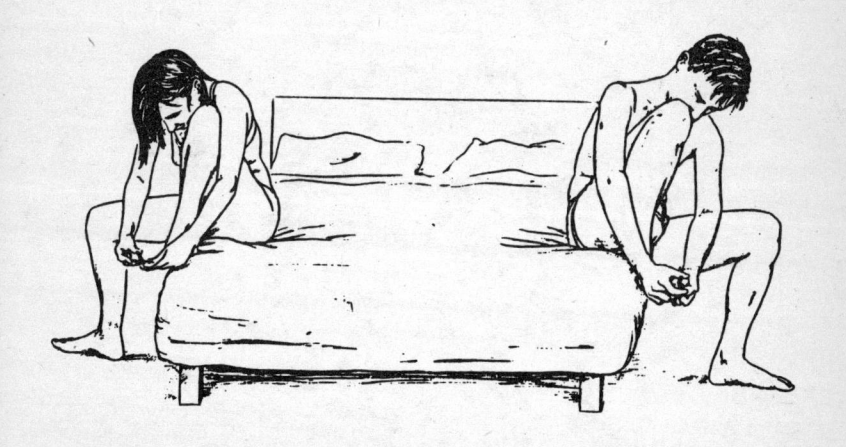

The act of celibacy. Two people completely at ease with each other in the perfect harmony of mutual celibacy

THE JOY OF CELIBACY

By now the celibate in you should be starting to assert itself. You no longer feel ashamed of sudden impulses to do a spot of gardening or crochet a scarf. A great weight has been lifted from your loins, you've learnt how not to enjoy sex and are ready to tarmac over the garden of earthly delights.

PREPARATION

Getting in Shape

As with any new activity you will need to train to get the most out of celibacy. A potential celibate partner will appreciate it if you've made the effort to get in shape. Below are some recommended exercises.

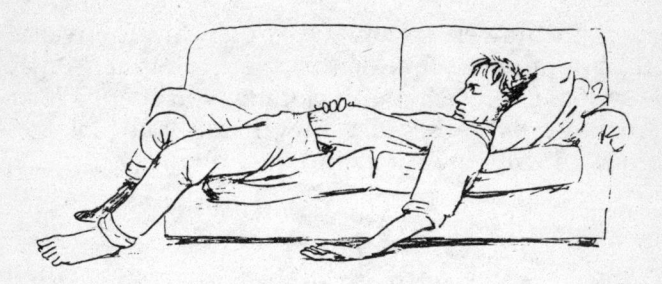

The sofa press. This is a particularly gruelling exercise as it can last anything up to three days

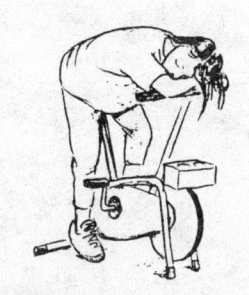

Be careful not to overdo it

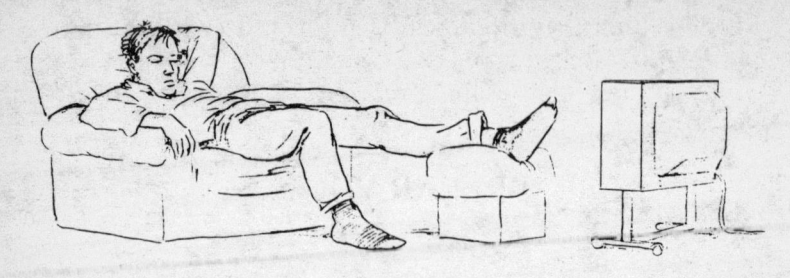

Leg extension – repeat several times a week

If you do not have access to special machines make the most of everyday opportunities – always take the lift instead of the stairs, take cabs where you used to walk and avoid all unnecessary movement.

Cultivating the Correct Look

The bottom drawer of your wardrobe can be invaluable when trying to put off sexual partners or attract someone more suitable. Those items of clothing you spent a fortune on but never wore because they made you look totally unattractive will now come into their own.

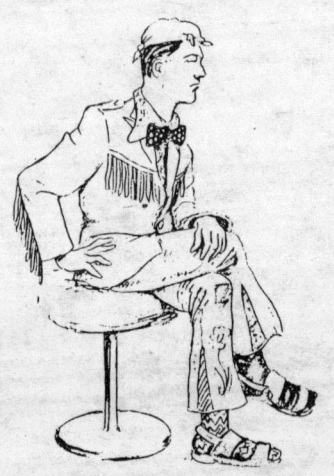

Mix styles. If possible stick to man-made fibres and make sure patterns clash

While bad taste is innate and cannot be taught, there are certain general principles one can follow.

Hair styling is equally important. Experiment with a comb and some gel to find your own personal worst style.

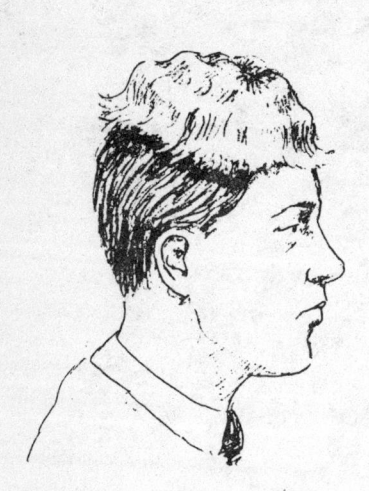

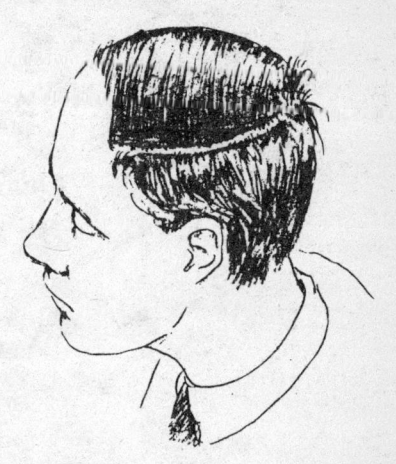

Make it look as though you're trying to cover up a bald patch

Dye half of hair a slightly different shade to enhance the effect

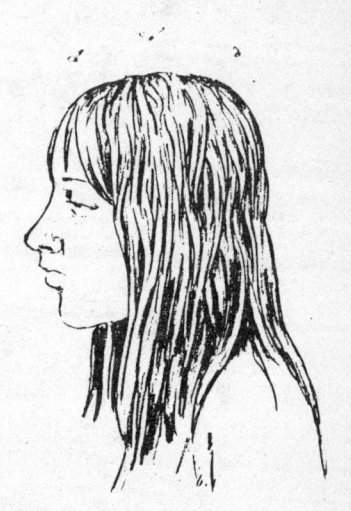

Don't wash your hair for a month

BEING CELIBATE FOR THE FIRST TIME

You've both got high expectations – you've heard and read so much about this moment that when it comes you're bound to be nervous about failing. Don't worry, however gauche and inept you are, as long as you don't have sex you will have succeeded. There will be plenty of time later to polish your performance.

Even if you know the person well, appealing to the celibate in them will feel like meeting them for the first time. You owe it to yourselves to try and make this a special occasion.

Setting the Scene

Music is a great inspiration. A brass band on tape, or if possible live in the room, has an invigorating and thoroughly non-sexual effect. It is difficult for conversation to become intimate if you are trying to bellow over the Huddersfield Brass Ensemble.

Well-chosen lighting can transform a seductive love-nest into a harsh and unforgiving laboratory. Install plenty of high-wattage sodium lamps and, of course, fluorescent tubes.

Children can create a useful disturbance and also serve to remind you of the awful consequences of sexual liaisons. Arm them with noisy battery-operated toys and make sure they are hungry and irritable. If you don't have a child of your own, you can borrow one for the night and earn yourself ten pounds into the bargain.

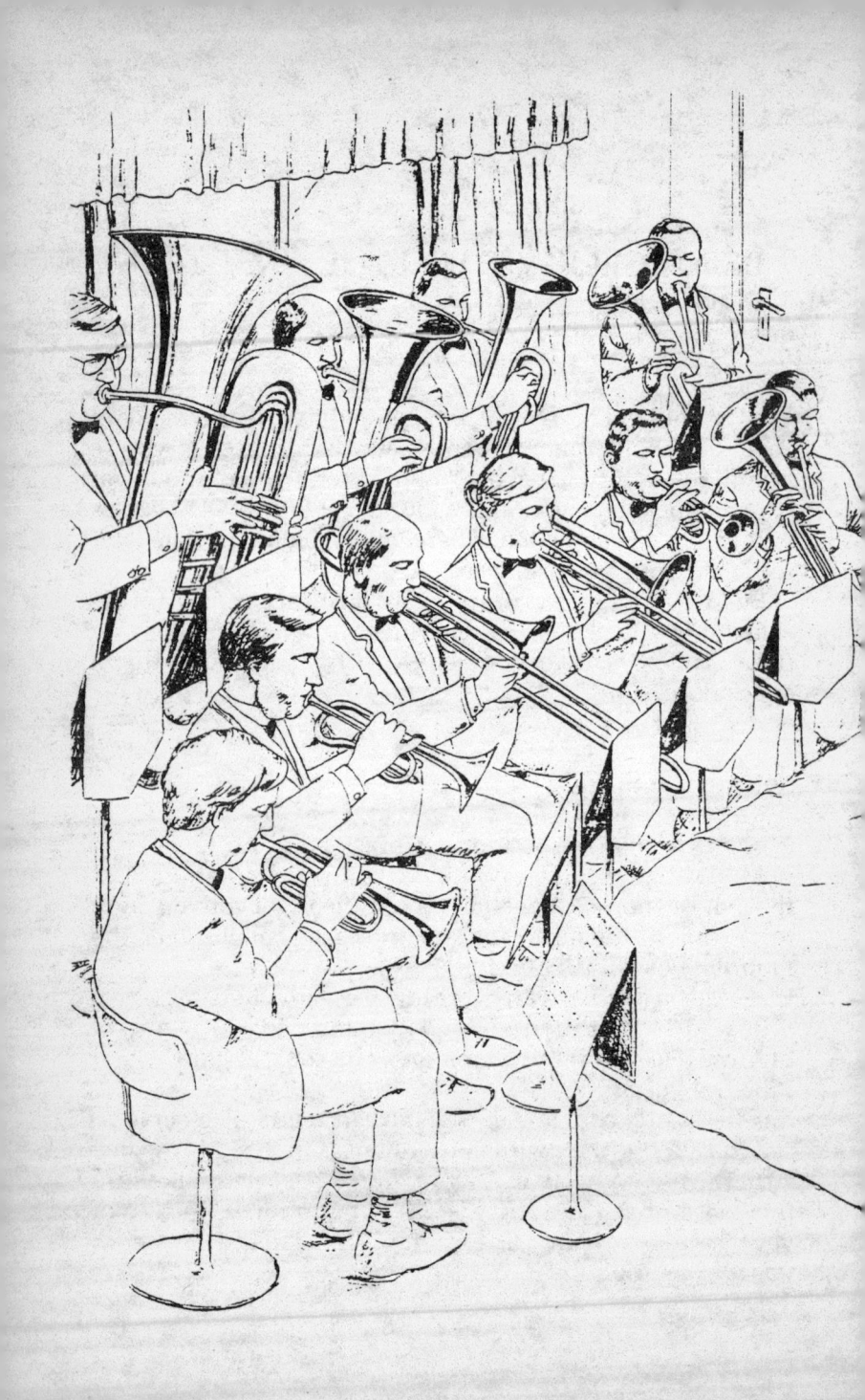

Your partner should now be in no doubt about your real intentions and you are ready to proceed to the next stage.

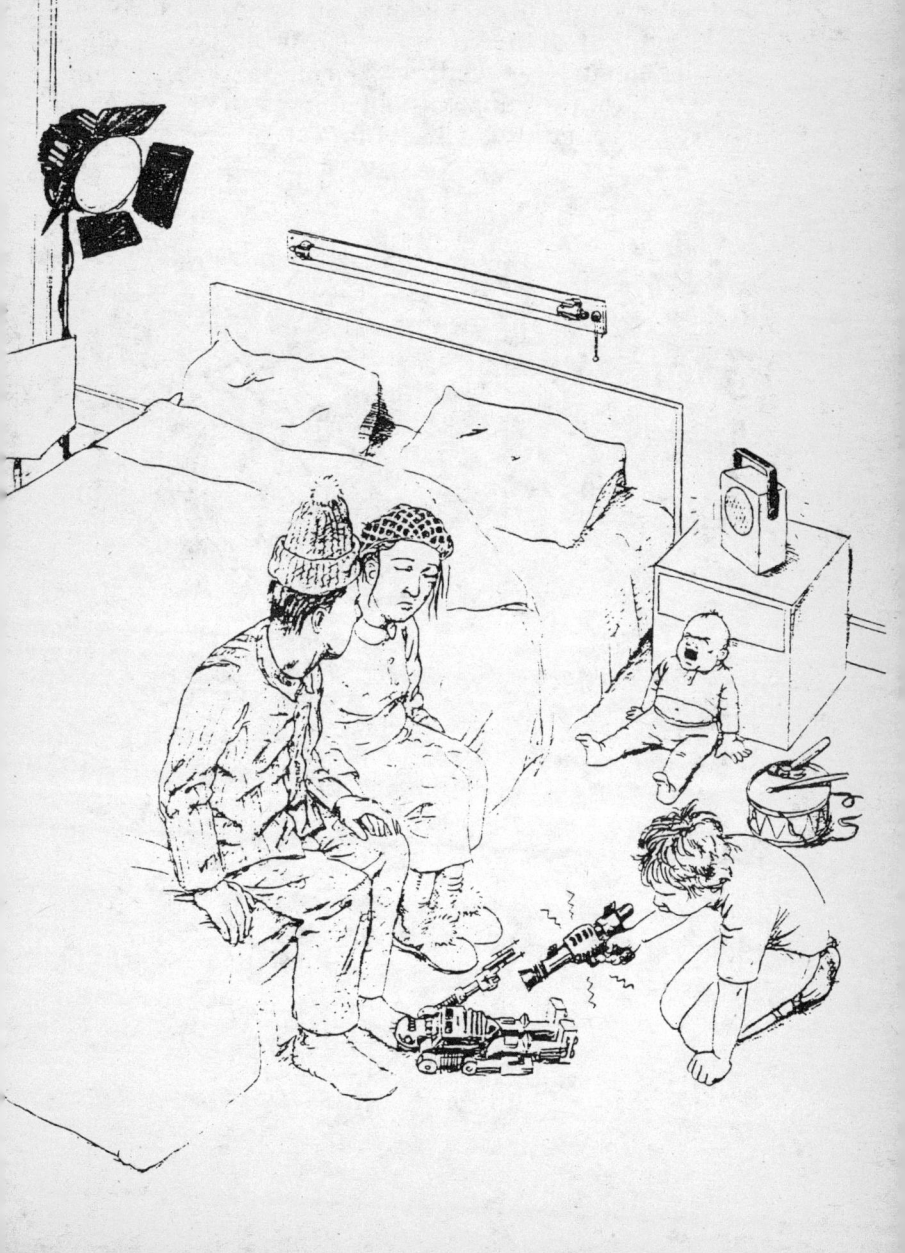

Celibate Foreplay

Any attempt to do without tactile sensations is dangerous at this point. Do not cut out nibbling, sucking and slurping altogether, but divert them to inanimate objects which you know will remain unmoved by your attentions. If your partner is reluctant or uncomprehending at first, *you* will have to show them the way. Let your imagination run riot!

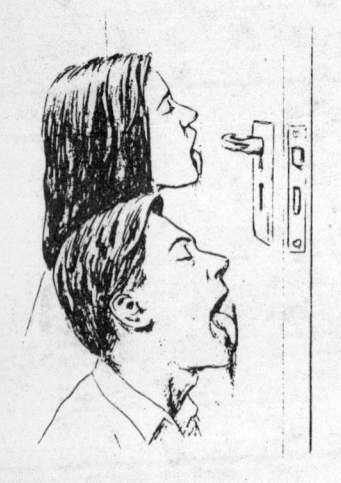

Give your door a tongue bath . . . take it in turns!

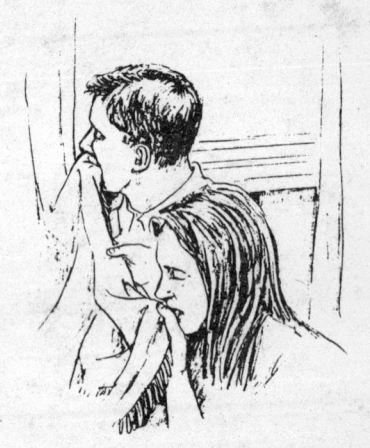

Tuning in to tassels and togs

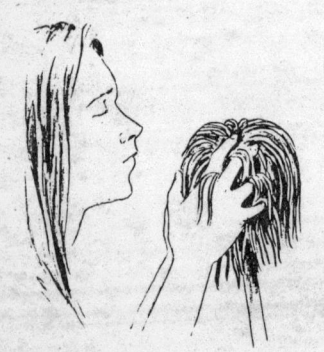

Run your fingers through a wet mop

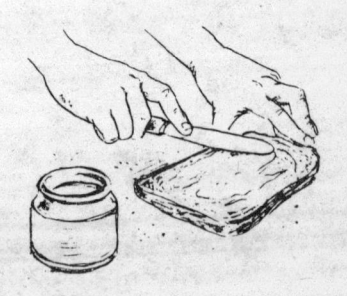

Try spreading peanut butter on toast for a change

Using Fantasies

Sit quietly with your partner and relax mentally to allow celibate thoughts to enter your head. An enjoyable experience in itself, this also serves to heighten anticipation. If you have a particularly celibate thought you may want to share it, especially if your partner is still struggling with semi-unerotic imagery.

Don't be ashamed if vivid celibate fantasies start flooding into your head, such as sleeping overnight at an airport, watching a video at a post office or surveying a house you don't intend to buy. A strong imagination can only help your relationship and you'll be limiting possibilities by keeping it to yourself. Your partner won't think less of you and will probably have had similar fantasies themselves.

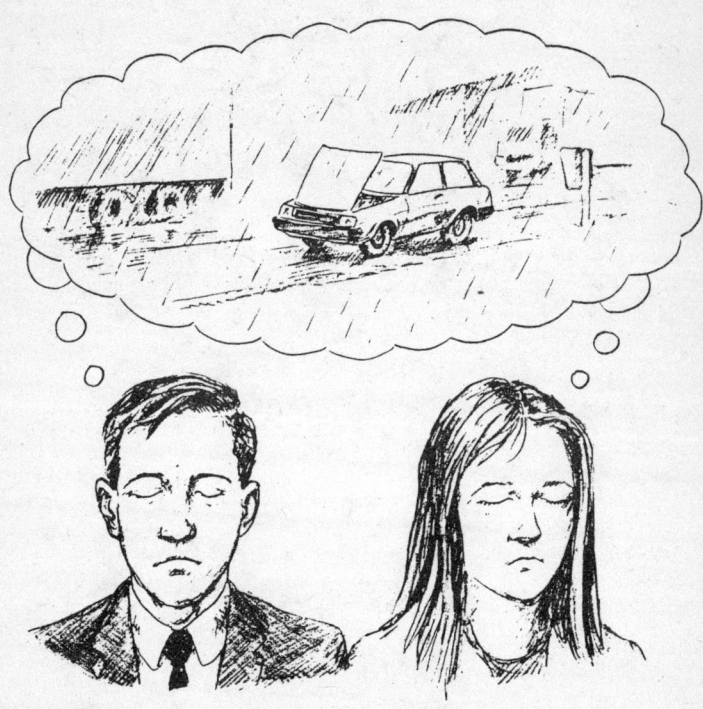

Waiting for the AA to turn up

Positions for Celibacy

How you most want to be celibate is entirely up to you. But the variety of positions you have to choose from is almost endless, ranging from basic to the exotic.

Note: many couples find a problem with lubrication. If so there is nothing to stop you offering each other a glass of water or even blackcurrant drink.

There are only two guidelines in good celibacy; don't do anything you really enjoy and find out your partner's needs and ignore them.

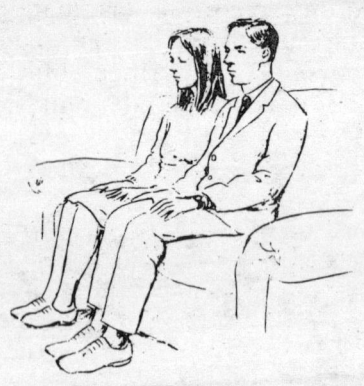

Missionary – the standard position that has served celibates well over the centuries. However many variations you try you're likely to come back to this well-tested favourite

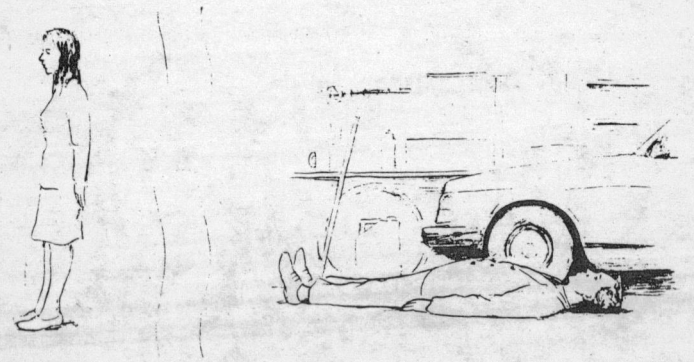

Against the wall – the woman props herself against the wall while the man lies on the garage floor (you may need cushions for this)

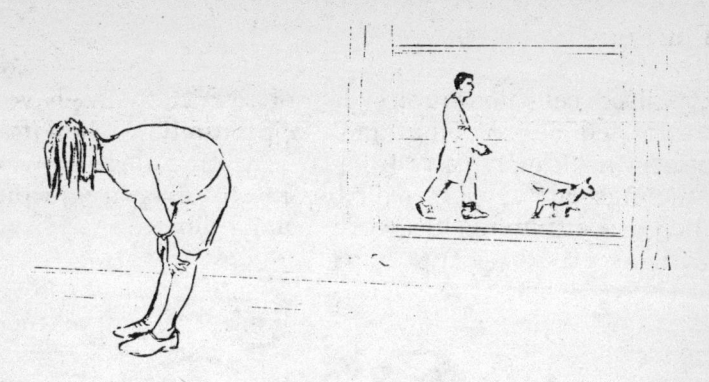

Doggie-fashion – the woman bends over while the man takes the dog for a walk

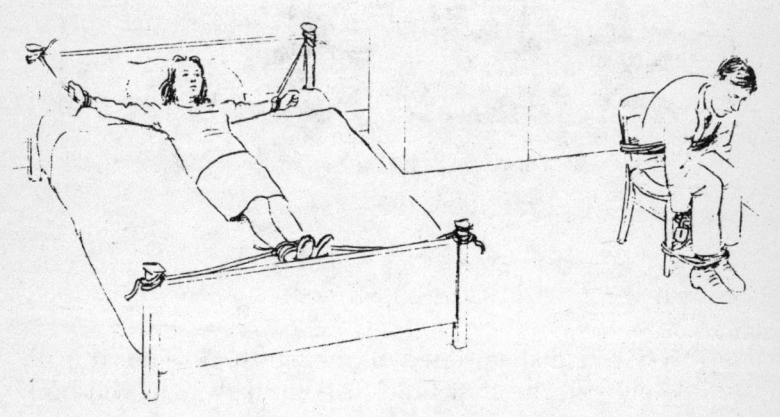

Bondage can offer a new dimension. After you've tied up your partner padlock yourself several feet away

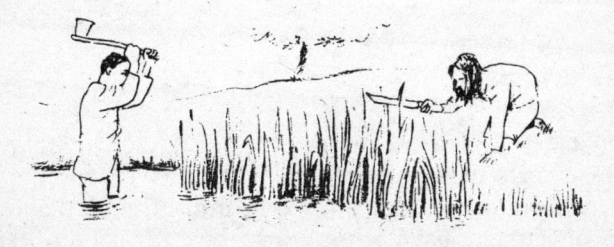

Splitting the reed – very popular in China and other parts of the Far East, this requires considerable physical strength and manual dexterity

37

Quickies

Practised celibate couples do not restrict themselves to prolonged sessions but grab opportunities when they arise. Inspiration can strike at any time – in between meetings, at the pub, over breakfast – even if you only have a few minutes it is worth being celibate.

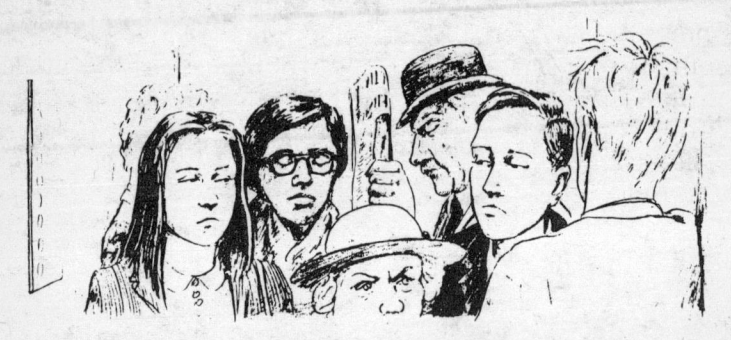

A crowded place can add an interesting element of risk

What if the Earth Starts to Move?

Don't be too disheartened if the earth doesn't remain completely still the first time. It is unlikely you will both feel the same level of indifference – truly mutual celibacy only comes with practice. At first you are both bound to make mistakes.

Mutual Celibacy

The best way to learn how to give someone the pleasures of celibacy is to watch them being celibate with themselves. No two individuals are celibate in quite the same way so it is important to learn what works best for each other.

When your partner is feeling particularly cold and indifferent sit quietly and note how they use their body, pay attention to the way they don't touch themselves, how they turn themselves off and prevent themselves feeling any sexual sensations. Later, you can be celibate while they watch.

After Celibacy

Some couples worry about going out after being celibate, convinced everyone will know what they've been up to. In fact one of the bonuses of celibacy is that very few people can tell the difference between someone who is celibate and someone who just happens not to be having sex. Even if they do they probably won't care.

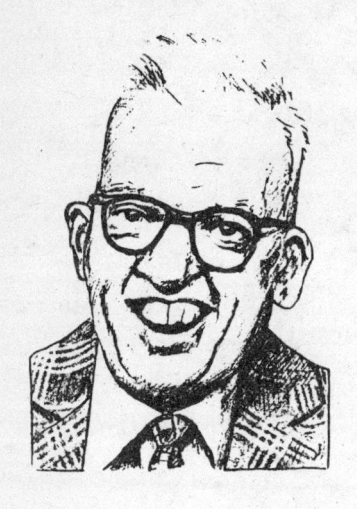

This person is not having sex.   *This person is being celibate.*

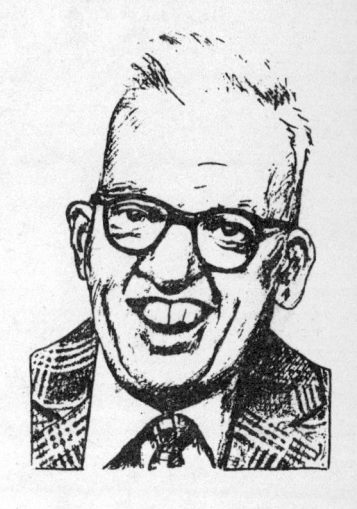

NB It is of course easier to spot a celibate man than a celibate woman

CELIBACY AND THE SINGLE PERSON

If you are a single person you will have spent years seeing everyone you meet as a potential sexual partner. Instead of undressing them in your imagination, try to visualise what they would look like with *more* clothes on. Picture them doing something particularly celibate, such as creosoting a rose trellis. As your fantasies change so gradually will your behaviour.

Making a Pig's Ear of It

The first step is to make a mess of any potentially sexual encounter – this is much easier then getting it right. Remember, a good non-sexual advance is the same as a bad sexual one. Inexperienced celibates can be awkward and ungainly, brushing past people instead of bumping into them and giving long sensuous kisses instead of wet, slobbery ones.

You will need a certain awareness and sensitivity to choose the most inappropriate moment to make a pass. Pay attention to the nature of the situation, choosing a moment when they are particularly engrossed in some other activity, such as changing lanes on a motorway, removing a splinter or when you are in front of the family, preferably at the funeral of a loved one. Timing is important: either make your move as soon as you meet someone or several years after they first showed interest.

Side Effects

One of the dangers of being a single celibate is that people may not be put off by your surliness, terrible dress sense and social ineptitude. They may see them as a challenge and try to break through to the 'real sexual you'. If this is the case you will have to take drastic measures: propose marriage and, if you are a woman, say you want to bear his children – this will put most people off.

Meeting Potential Partners

Unfortunately, there are no hard and fast rules for meeting suitable partners. Some people are just born less charismatic and there is no point resenting this, you simply have to learn to make the least of your sexual magnetism.

The prospect of meeting someone suitable may seem daunting at first. However, the chances of finding someone who is at least basically incompatible are very high. One way is to take a nightclass in a subject in which you have no interest, this will ensure you meet a number of people with whom you have nothing in common.

How do I tell when Someone Doesn't Want to Have Sex with me?

You will need to be extremely sensitive to suggestion here, as the signs celibates give out are not always obvious. If someone doesn't look round when you enter the room or show any inclination to talk to you, then they are telling you in no uncertain terms that they want to be celibate, but not everyone is that forthright. Lapses in conversation and vacant looks can speak volumes. A yawn back across a crowded room can be all that you need.

Is it Right to be Celibate on a First Date?

Some people may want to be celibate with you but not on the first date – if you think they're worth it you'll just have to be patient, after all there is more to a relationship than just not-having sex. It can be counterproductive to push people into unwanted celibacy. It won't do you any harm to wait, indeed many couples who are celibate the first time, quickly tire of the novelty and slip back into sex.

Making a Celibate Advance

A celibate pass means making it absolutely clear you don't want to have sex with someone. Try to find yourself in potentially provocative situations and then show complete indifference.
Other tried and tested methods:

Go on a long drive in the country and completely fail to run out of petrol or break down at any point.

If you are in a pub together, try spilling beer over your trousers and then rush off home to put them in the wash.

At the cinema, make sure your partner is comfortably settled in the back row of the stalls – then go and sit in the upper circle.

You can easily tell if your advances have been reciprocated – your partner should remain completely still and passive. A hot tongue in the ear, on the other hand, does not augur well – you may have to write this one off to experience.

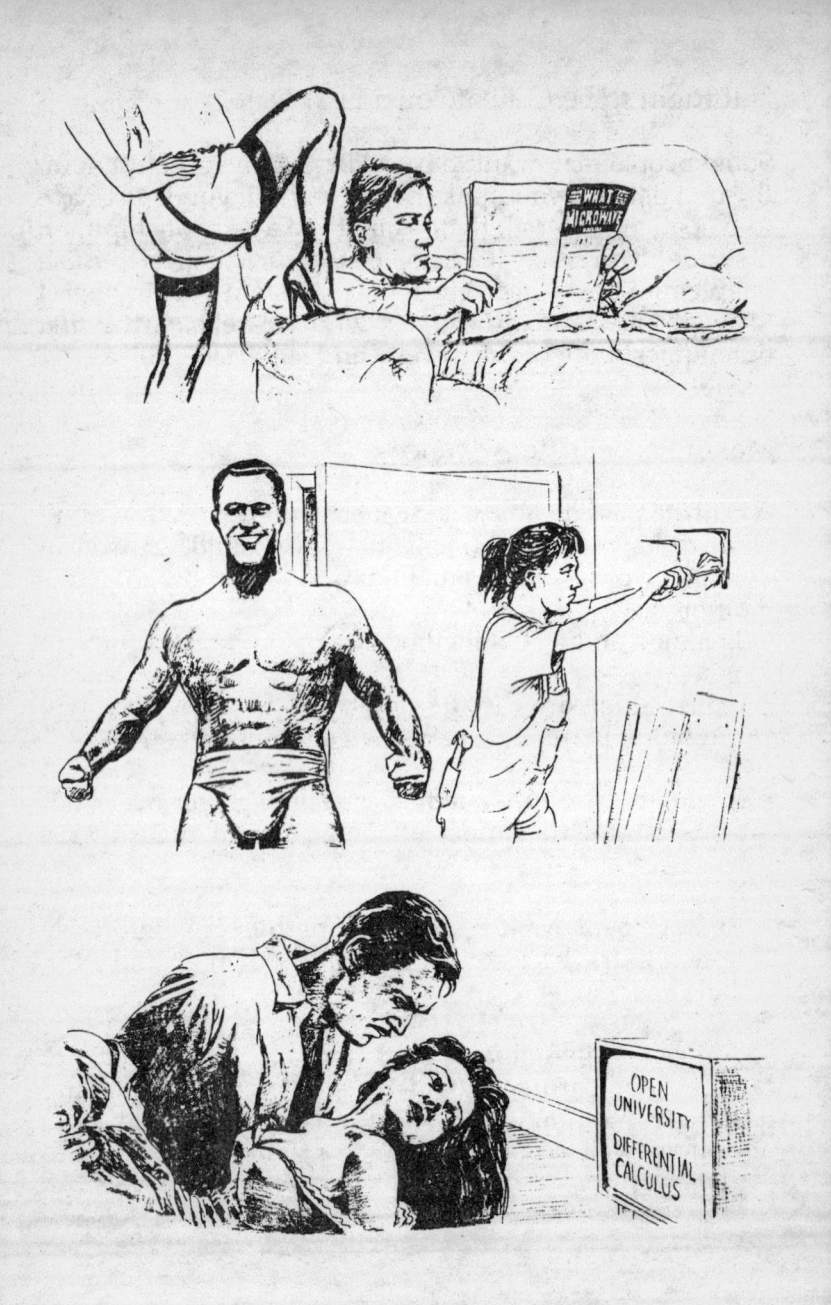

Putting it About

There's nothing wrong with cultivating a string of casual celibate encounters as long as you both feel the same way and no one gets hurt. But be sure you can handle the consequences of not sleeping with someone you may never see again. Short-term affairs sometimes feel superficial but they will stand you in good stead if you ever want to take the plunge and settle down. Few people subscribe to the old idea of keeping yourself for one celibate partner, indeed many prefer someone with experience.

Jealousy

Only the most uptight people are likely to be jealous of other celibate relationships. It is healthy to discuss past celibate affairs openly but if your partner starts asking who you were celibate with last night, it may be time to move on and not have sex with someone else.

THE FACTS ABOUT CELIBACY

A great deal of mystery and superstition still surrounds the true nature of celibacy. Prejudice and misunderstanding exist even today because people rely on misinformation and are afraid to ask questions. It's strange that while most schoolchildren are well informed about the G-spot and the difference between the labia majora and labia minora, they know nothing about the non-erogenous zones.

Certain areas of the body are definitely less sexy than others and are thus less likely to respond to stimulation. As a non-sexual being these are the parts that should interest you most. Study the illustrations below and concentrate your efforts on the areas marked. Although it cannot be guaranteed they will not arouse, they are safer than a good many others.

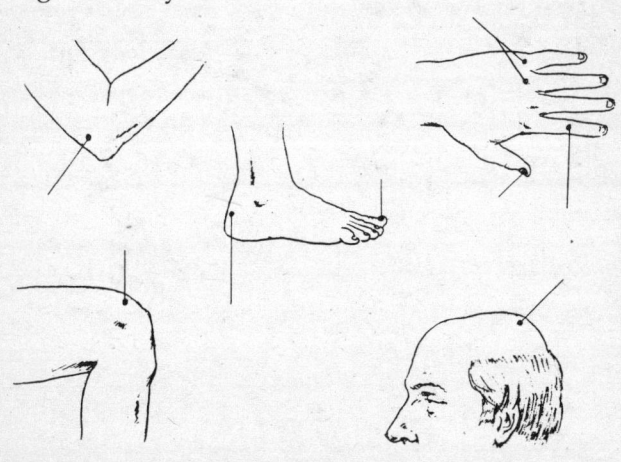

People who have already discovered that certain parts of their bodies are less responsive than others are often worried that their non-sexual organs are not of the 'correct' size. There is no correct size. With feet, for example, anything between a size 5 and 9 is perfectly adequate. Enlargement rarely works and can be dangerous – the special lotions, creams and vacuum gadgets are no more than gimmicks.

The C-Spot

The ultimate non-erogenous zone is the elusive C-spot – the one part of your anatomy that is completely sexually inert. The exact position of this spot differs from person to person.

Locating the C-spot is of fundamental importance. Although time-consuming and arousing, with perseverance and a cold-douche at hand it can be found. Once identified it will be a source of unfulfilment for many years.

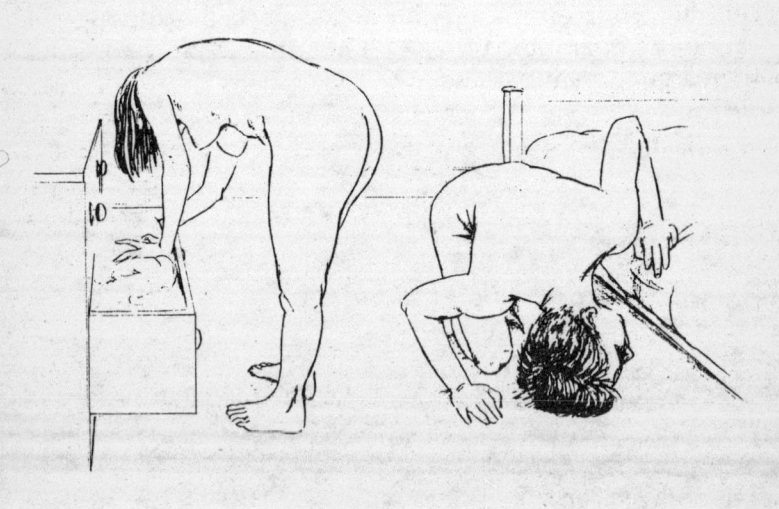

Looking for the C-Spot

What Happens During Celibacy?

The obvious answer is nothing, but this is not nearly the whole picture. You still at first notice a general numbness come over you, a desire to do very little, not to move or stir yourself at all unless to make a cup of tea or turn on the television. There is a decrease in the blood flow to most organs, the body relaxes, the skin goes flabby, the eyes feel heavy and there is a strong urge to sleep – an experience you may well want to repeat soon afterwards. Really good celibacy should leave you uncertain whether you've had it at all.

Post-Celibate Blues

This refers to the feeling of emptiness and disappointment which often follows celibacy. This is only natural and will pass after a few months. Indeed, as you progress you will learn to cherish these feelings as the just rewards of celibacy.

Homo-Celibacy

In some cultures celibacy between people of the same sex is still a crime, in others it is widely accepted. Statistics show that ninety per cent of men have, at one time or another, been celibate with other men. The percentage may be even higher for women.

Contrary to popular belief, being celibate with the same sex differs very little from 'hetero-celibacy'. There are no special techniques and the feelings of uninterest are very similar. Indeed many long-term celibates would claim that you cannot lead a fully satisfying celibate life without exploring all possibilities with both sexes.

The Celibate Teenager

Adolescence is a distressing time when many people first discover their celibate inclinations. Teenagers are often ashamed of how much of their day they spend thinking about celibacy – there seems to be nothing else on their minds. This is quite normal – the average male has celibate thoughts once every two minutes.

It is also a time when your body starts to play strange tricks on you. Just when you thought your hormones were on your side, giving you puppy-fat and acne, you suddenly wake up with clear skin and nubile good looks. Although this can ruin your confidence at the time, bear in mind that this is only a stage – it is almost certain you will never look this good again. In a few short years gravity will take hold of those firm thighs, age will etch its way into your face and you can relax in the knowledge the great sag has begun.

There can also be a great social pressure to have sex, usually from parents and teachers. If you are forced by your school to attend classes on cunnilingus and fellatio you might like to form your own celibate club where you can discuss gardening or other topics of interest.

Young people often desperately fear parental disapproval and keep their celibacy to themselves, confining it to locked bathrooms and the safety of their bedrooms. Reactionary parents find it difficult to accept that their off-spring have 'chosen' to be celibate. They will be disappointed if you come home with a partner, ask for separate rooms and then don't creep along the corridor in the middle of the night. If you are concerned to initiate your parents without embarrassment, casually leave this book on their bed.

ADJUSTING TO CELIBATE LIFE

Coming Out

Should I tell people I'm celibate? It very much depends on the situation. Sometimes it is inappropriate to announce you are celibate, such as at a dinner party, while on others, at a sales conference for example, it is wise to let people know as early as possible or you might end up being invited to the type of party which could set back your plans by several weeks.

Stamina

Early on you may find that you can only be celibate once or twice a night, though the time it takes to 'recover' varies with age and gender. Don't be intimidated by claims of celibate prowess – it is not the number of times you manage it but the quality of each encounter that is important. Celibate stamina only comes with practice – the more you don't do it the better you'll get.

Diet

A change in your eating habits will help. As your sexual desire begins to wain you will naturally opt for new types of food. No longer will you require fresh fruit, vegetables and lean meat; instead you should switch to a more 'celibate' diet of chocolates, chips and fried food.

Sex Toys

Old sex toys need not be thrown out – with a little imagination they can be adapted to your new interests. You can spend an enjoyable evening together sewing up your crotchless pants; a vibrator makes an eye-catching drinks mixer, while an old pair of French knickers easily becomes a serviceable grow-bag.

Alternatively you can take your vibrators, dildos and bondage shorts down to the local Oxfam shop – they will find a good home for them and help the underprivileged at the same time. You can specify where you want your vibrator to go – perhaps the Sudan or Ethiopia.

Withdrawal Symptoms

At some point, all celibates can expect to suffer from an attack of sudden sexuality. Some are overwhelmed by a wave of involuntary randiness, others simply do not feel like celibacy. This can be for any number of reasons; you may be too tired or simply have had a surfeit of celibacy in recent weeks. The best advice in these situations is to stick it out and sit on it. It will soon pass and your old celibate feelings stir into action again.

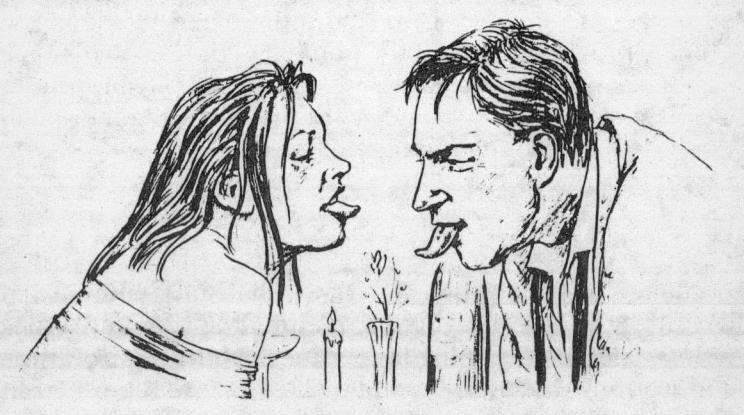

Sometimes you're just not in the mood for celibacy

Erections

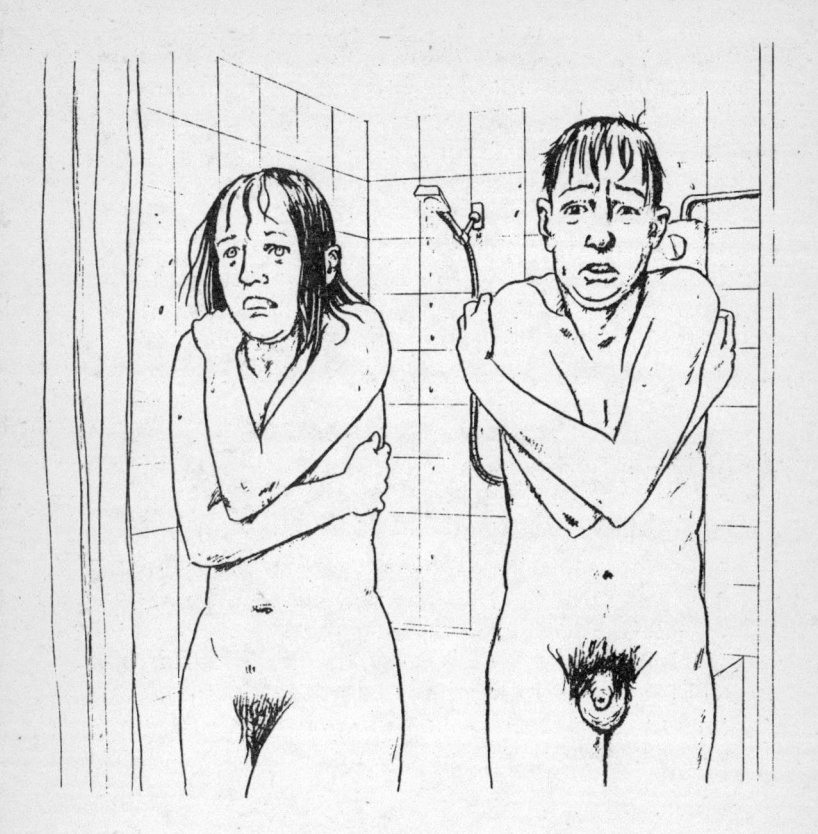

Ready for celibacy after a bracing cold shower

It can be worrying when your penis completely fails to be limp but seems to take on a life of its own, making it very hard for you and your partner to fully enjoy celibacy together. You may resort to drugs, alcohol or even try dunking it in a pitcher of ice cold water, but the fact is that no artificial aids are going to revive a flagging relationship. The real problem is that you've allowed your celibate life to become tired and routine.

SPICING UP YOUR CELIBATE LIFE

It is important to keep your celibacy alive and interesting. Most celibate relationships fail because the couple get stuck in a rut. The more celibate you are the more experimental you can afford to be. Don't restrict yourself to the bed. You can be celibate anywhere, at any time: be adventurous – try it in public, on a bus, in the park, even in front of unsuspecting friends.

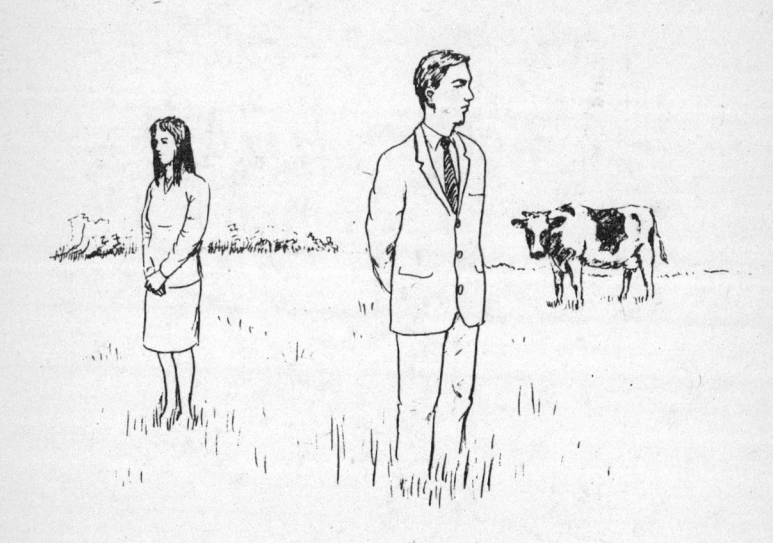

Kinky Celibacy

Some celibates find they have unusual desires which can't be catered for inside their normal relationship. These special needs have been well documented and it is unlikely yours is any more shocking than anyone else's. Over the last few thousand years people have been celibate with just about everything. Here are a few of the more common variations:

Group Celibacy

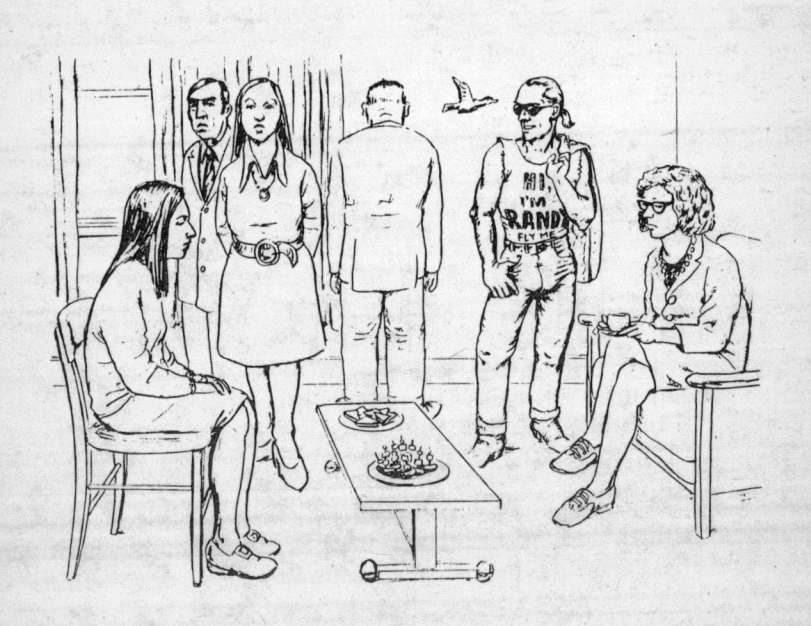

You may like to liven up your celibacy by joining like-minded celibates for group sessions. This sometimes reinvigorates stagnant relationships and can certainly provide a couple with lots of new and useful information on non-sexual behaviour. There is nothing wrong with sharing your celibacy with others, though regular partners can become jealous. If either of you is reluctant or can't handle the idea, steer well clear.

If, however, you've both talked it over and are sure you don't mind sharing, the best way of meeting 'swinging' celibates is through a whist-drive. But beware of the occasional non-celibate slipping into your midst and ruining the whole thing.

Animals

You might have sometimes wondered what it was like to be celibate with a dog or a horse. Similar to human celibacy in most ways, it has the added attraction that the animal will remain completely oblivious. Provided you stick to its natural habitat it is unlikely to do the animal any harm. The incidence of this form of celibacy is particularly high amongst pet-owners.

Incest

Although a taboo subject, society has become increasingly aware of celibacy within the family. Statistics show that most people do at one time or another harbour celibate thoughts about parents, children or siblings.

Fetishes

A person may feel especially unaroused by certain items of clothing and accessories.

A mild form of fetishism is perfectly acceptable, but there can be a danger of it becoming obsessional. In extreme cases the celibate substitutes the clothing for the person themself. This is *not* advised as it can result in being celibate with a rack of Marks and Spencers anoraks.

Uniform fetishism probably goes back to childhood

when infants were introduced to the idea of not having sex with people in uniform. It can have long term effects, with many people wanting to be celibate with such figures as vicars, nuns and policemen.

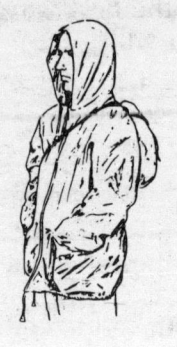

A Millets cagoul and a Karimor bag almost universally trigger a celibate response

Role Playing

Acting out fantasies can be an important element in any successful relationship and is fine as long as each partner is happy with their role and you both know when to stop.

Don't be surprised if you are required to dress up as a museum attendant and stand in an art gallery for an afternoon. But if your partner asks you to take the job full-time, they may be becoming obsessive and you'll have to draw the line.

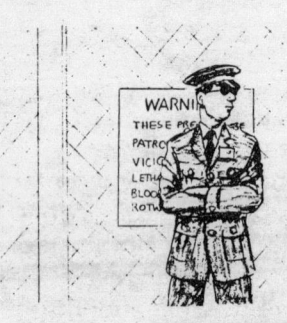

Acting out the Security Guard Fantasy

Power games are another variation. You can take it in turns to dominate each other, one partner pretending to be reluctant while the other forces them to have celibacy. Such games are perfectly all right as long as they are not mistaken for the real thing.

Voyeurism

Some people enjoy watching strangers being celibate. Again, this is quite harmless as long as it does not replace the celibate act altogether.

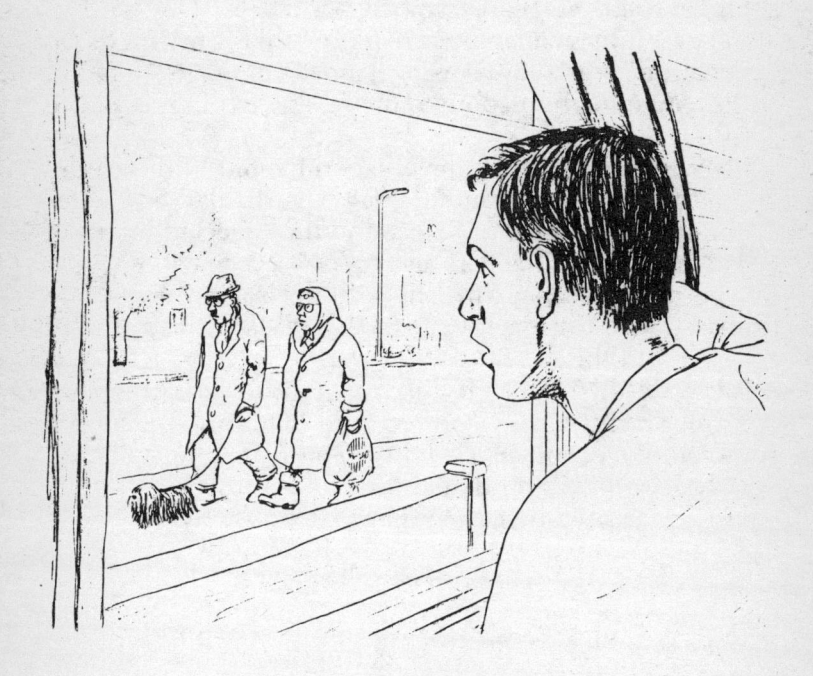

Phones

The phone has introduced a whole new range of celibate fetishes, from developing an intimate relationship with the handset itself, through to making celibate calls to complete strangers and chatting to them about the weather. If you receive an unwelcome 'clean' call try to appear shocked, if you seem bored this will only excite and encourage them.

Pornography

There is a vast amount of specialist literary and visual material available to inspire the celibate. Couples sometimes use it to give their relationship a boost, singles to satisfy themselves temporarily. Statistics have shown that a higher percentage of women are affected by verbal/literary material whilst men are more visually oriented. An extract from a car manual will get most women in the mood while a man might respond more readily to pictures of fire doors.

Many literary figures have experimented with writing of this kind, most unintentionally. Particular favourites include Joyce's *Finnegan's Wake* and the collected works of Hermann Hesse. There are also specialist magazines which can be purchased in virtually any newsagent if you are prepared to ask discreetly, including *What Microwave?*, *The Engineer* and the *TV Times*.

It can be distressing to discover that your partner has a secret stash of hard-core celibate literature, such as a complete collection of *Concrete Pilings*, making you feel deeply inadequate and insecure. It is probably best to confront them with your find and discuss why they need this kind of material.

Professional Celibates

Some celibates, or those in particularly satisfying sexual partnerships, may have latent celibate desires which can only be satisfied outside their normal relationship. They may seek special celibate services, often paying for the privilege. It is fairly simple to get into contact with someone who will provide this sort of assistance – in most towns and cities there is an area well-known for celibate encounters, such as a public library, town hall or tax office. Alternatively, newspapers carry classified advertisements offering celibate contacts. These are usually thinly disguised as motoring advertisements or announcements of jumble sales.

Breaking Up

Despite all your efforts your celibate relationship may just be beyond repair. You should not feel guilty about this. Perhaps you are just too compatible, too sexually well-suited. In such cases you will have to take the difficult decision to break up and find someone whom you find less attractive.

If you are worried about your partner's reaction, remember: the truth may not hurt them as much as you think. They have, after all, at least been trying not to get involved with you. You may find that when you finally pluck up the courage to let them know you no longer want to be celibate they tell you they were unaware they were having a relationship with you anyway.

Experiment with some of these useful phrases:

You're just not the sort of person I can be celibate with.
I just don't think we're incompatible.
You're more like a lover to me.
I'm sure you'll find there are lots of people who don't want to sleep with you – you're a very unattractive person.

THE FUTURE

When all that remains of your sex life is a distant memory and a few stains on your carpet, you will finally be enjoying the fruits of celibacy. All your work and sacrifice will have paid off and you will wonder how you ever managed not to do without it. Your only remaining fear may be about the future: will celibacy become more difficult, will people still want to be celibate with you in fifteen years' time?

The good news is the quality of your celibate life can only get better with age. You have years and years to cultivate and refine your celibacy in the sure knowledge that your capacity for it will only improve. Most people reach their celibate peak somewhere in their sixties and rarely go down hill from there. You may even be lucky enough to die in the act of celibacy – the most dignified way to end a celibate life.

JOE DA VINCI

THE BOOK OF BOTTOMS

HERE IT IS BOTTOM WATCHERS – YOUR VERY OWN HANDBOOK!

Despair no more, bottom-fanciers, your time has come! Expert clunologist Joe Da Vinci has compiled *the* definitive guide to the wonderful world of the rear end. Learn all about:

- ★ Bottom Spotting For Beginners
- ★ The Ten Top Tushes of All Time – & The Ten Most Tasteless Tails
- ★ Shave 'n Paint Parties
- ★ Bottom Maintenance
- ★ Take The Clunology Quiz
- ★ Learn To Play Pucker Power

And hundred more facts, games, pictures and trivia. Hours of fun for the bottom enthusiast inside all of us!

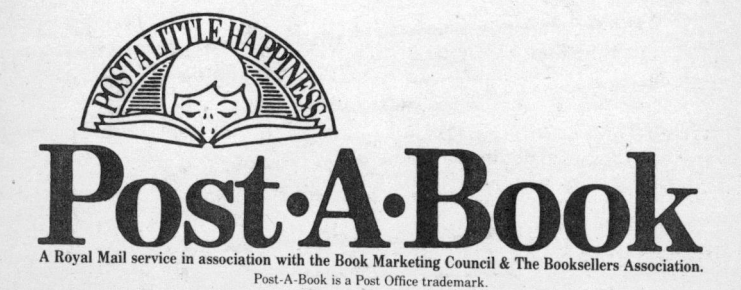

Post·A·Book

A Royal Mail service in association with the Book Marketing Council & The Booksellers Association.
Post-A-Book is a Post Office trademark.

MORE HUMOUR TITLES AVAILABLE FROM HODDER AND STOUGHTON PAPERBACKS

JOE DA VINCI
☐ 50810 2 The Book of Bottoms £2.99

DAVID RENWICK
☐ 50809 9 But I Digress £2.50

RONNIE BARKER
☐ 50813 7 It's Hello From Him £2.99

STEVE WRIGHT
☐ 49474 8 It's Another True Story £2.50

DEREK NIMMO
☐ 43072 9 Not In Front of the Servants £1.99
☐ 41537 1 Oh, Come On All Ye Faithful £1.95

All these books are available at your local bookshop or newsagent, or can be ordered direct from the publisher. Just tick the titles you want and fill in the form below.

Prices and availability subject to change without notice.

HODDER AND STOUGHTON PAPERBACKS, P.O. Box 11, Falmouth, Cornwall.

Please send cheque or postal order, and allow the following for postage and packing:

U.K. – 55p for one book, plus 22p for the second book, and 14p for each additional book ordered up to a £1.75 maximum.

B.F.P.O. and EIRE – 55p for the first book, plus 22p for the second book, and 14p per copy for the next 7 books, 8p per book thereafter.

OTHER OVERSEAS CUSTOMERS – £1.00 for the first book, plus 25p per copy for each additional book.

NAME ....

ADDRESS ....

....